The Things We've Done During The Pandemic For Fun, So Can You!

We say Ma, Grandma, Nana

KEON HINDS, SIAHNA WALKER, SAKYLA WALKER & SYDNIA WALKER

The Things We've Done During The Pandemic For Fun, So Can You!
Copyright © 2021 by Keon Hinds, Siahna Walker, Sakyla Walker, Sydnia Walker

All rights reserved. No part of this publication may be reproduced, distributed, or transmitted in any form or by any means, including photocopying, recording, or other electronic or mechanical methods, without the prior written permission of the author, except in the case of brief quotations embodied in critical reviews and certain other non-commercial uses permitted by copyright law.

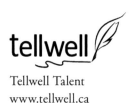

Tellwell Talent
www.tellwell.ca

ISBN
978-0-2288-6158-4 (Paperback)

Dedicated to our love ones, forever in our hearts.
R.I.P. Love Always!

Father- Winston/ pops

Grandma- Anna May

Brothers- Dennis & Donnie

Cousin/Sister-Pam

Nephew- William

God Son- TJ

Aunts-Lillian, Maryann, Dutches

Uncle-Junior

Cousins-Darran & Tiffany

Sakyla Walker, Siahna Walker,
Keon Hinds Walker, and Sydnia Walker

The things we've done during the pandemic for fun: so can you!

(We Call her Grandma/Ma, Nana)

Starting the day with joy, sets the mood. The love of having grandchildren is the sunshine of joy. The time is shared with love, teaching, encouraging social skills, learning skills, and values & morals that will remain within a child.

It is indeed incredible to understand the concept of time spend with children. Family plays a major role in one's life. Encouraging a child to reach beyond what they believe, allows them to reach their goals, dreams, and imagination of making all designs and desirable events that carry into their older years. One must be open to the creativity that each child brings fourth.

Taking unexpected time with grandchildren and other children to show how pictures can say a thousand words. Not planned, but just on a regular day or it can sometimes be planned. Taking time in the house or outside to do whatever comes to mind. Such as,

- walking to the store

- Riding to the store on the bike

- Teaching the children how to cook

- Play board games

- Helping with homework

- Drawing

- Making cup cakes

- Riding on rides

- Making up your own games

Kids will learn and grow in a great way; when they feel loved and connected. My point is, anytime you choose whatever you choose is a thing; which is a love thing. Whatever you may have around the house, it's about making the best time out of anytime. This makes the best time for laughing, learning, and growing. It's the ideas that's creates new thoughts of what else to do. Try it!

Every day is a new day for learning, even if it's through fun. Yes, kids will say-oh boy, we have to write, but the key is making games out of learning. During this process of learning/fun, the kids will totally forget they are learning. It is imperative to understand each child concept of thinking being every child has a different personality. Therefore, it is indeed a blessing to be able to understand each child needs. So, In the process of my grandchildren, expressing their feelings and thoughts of each picture of family members, they will go through each picture with stickers, and designs or whatever comes to mind. Grandchildren are a blessing; it is the foundation of values and morals that reflects on who we all are as individuals. This allows room to a great journey of success.

- Dr. Seuss. "The more that you read the more things you will know the more that you learn the more places you'll go."

Taking time out with the kids during the pandemic helped them to become more active around the house. Also, allowed them to express how they missed their peers and teachers in the school setting. However, they made the best of it with activities home. They Shared pictures of the past & present events, outdoor and indoor experiences through pictures. Pictures are expressed through so many lenses. They look at the pictures and articulate how their auntie, uncle cousins, God brother, Grandma, ma, and Nana made them feel or how they just like expressing what they were doing that day.

We leave space to ask you, how do you feel about the whole process of the pandemic and wearing a mask? Because knowing each child, helps with understanding their change of patterns with eating, sleeping, interacting with peers, and school work.

Overall, we as a family; would like to say thank you, for taking a journey through our peer support team work. We love having all types of activities, so we hope what we shared with you, will help you to do any activities you choose to do around your house.

At the bottom is a space to share your ideas. Also, what do you think is a good activity to do at your home or outside?

Just have fun, whatever you choose to do.

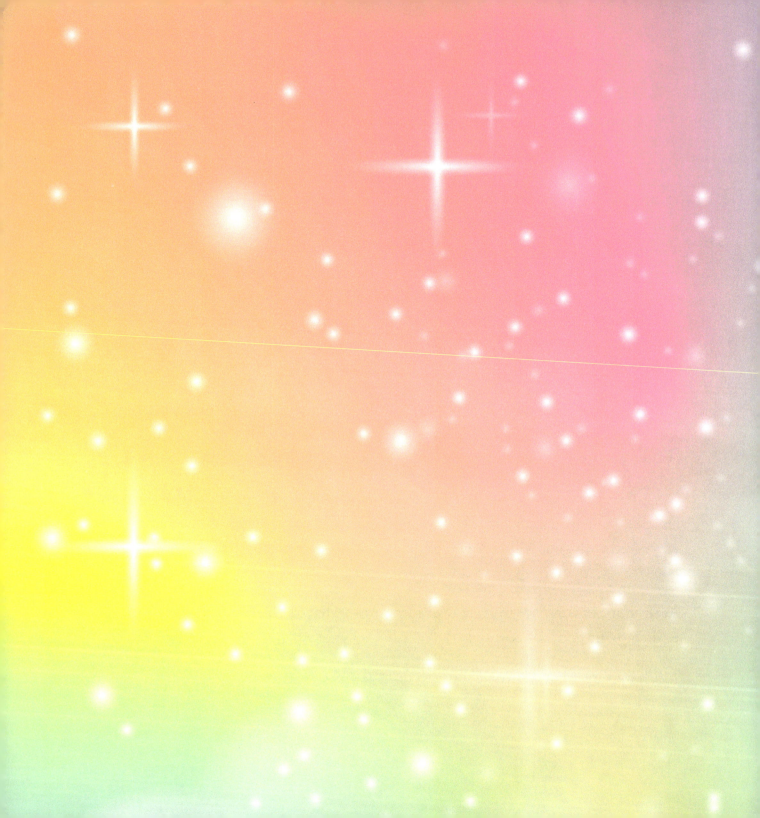

Birthdays

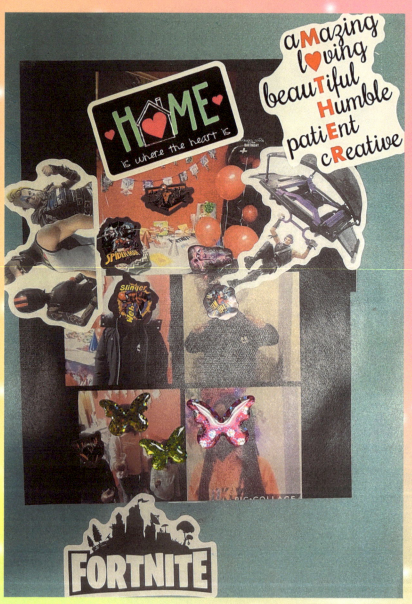

When is your birthday?
More birthday time.

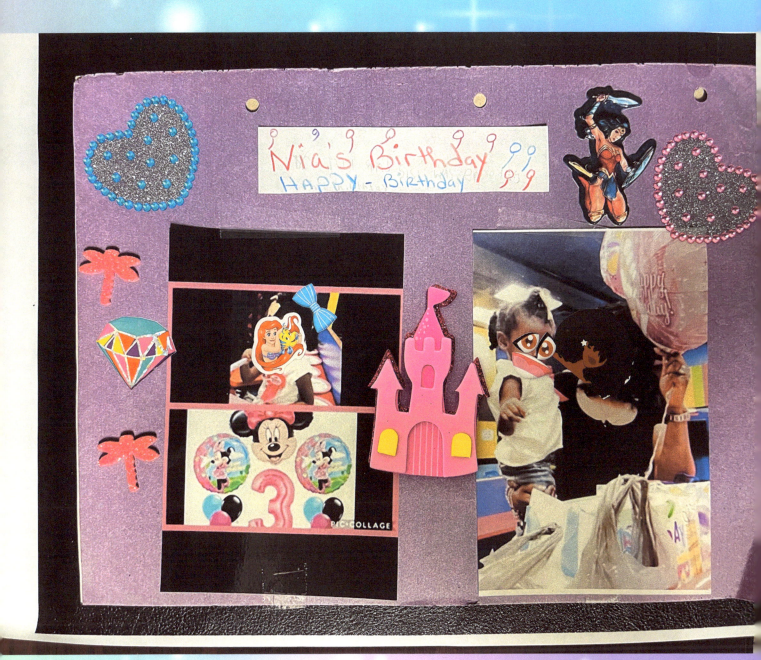

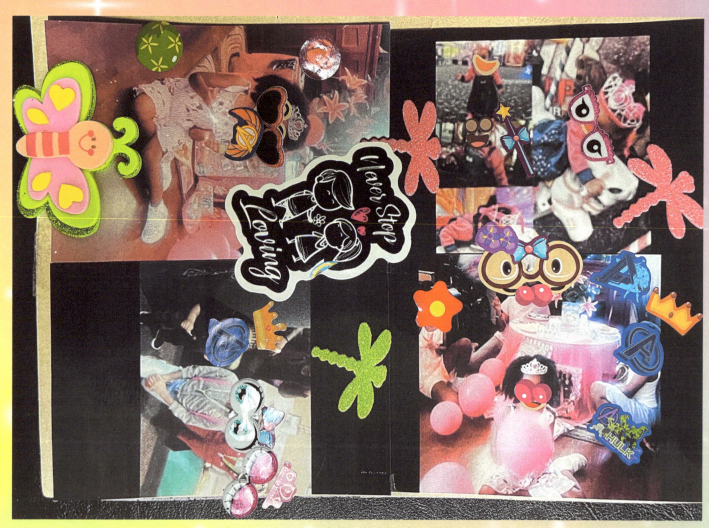

I love Birthday time. Do you like Birthday time?

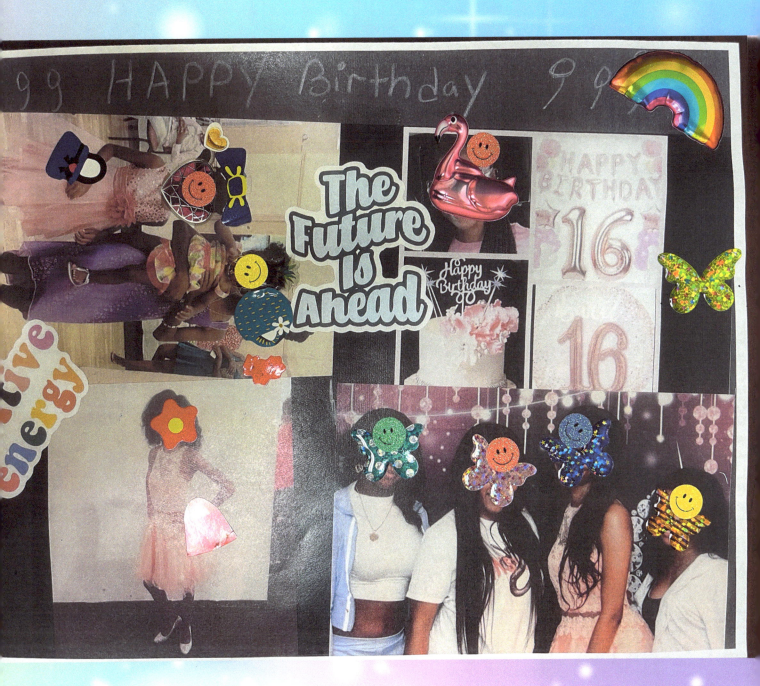

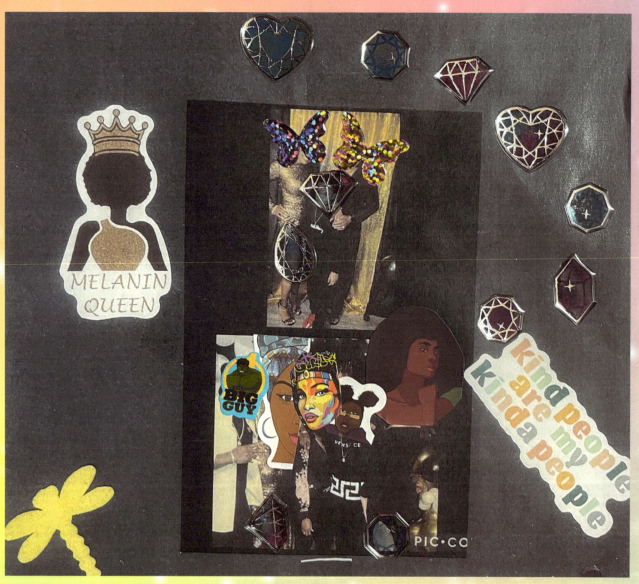

Happy Birthday!

Would you like t o say Happy Birthday?

Christmas

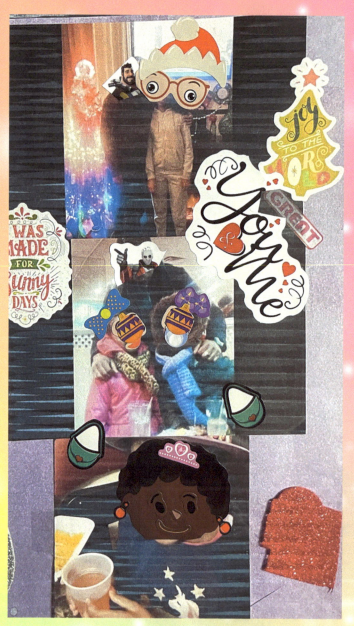

A nice day out side to have a nice day.

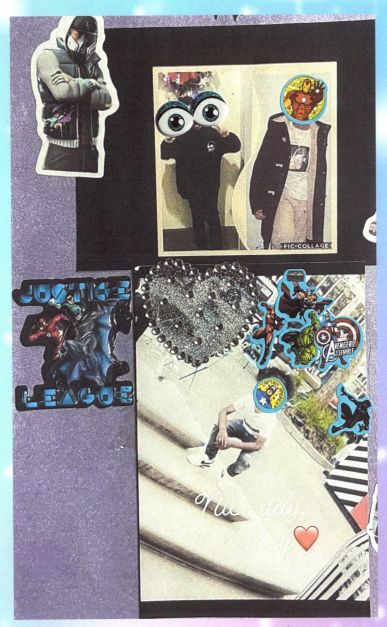

A nice day out side to have a nice day.

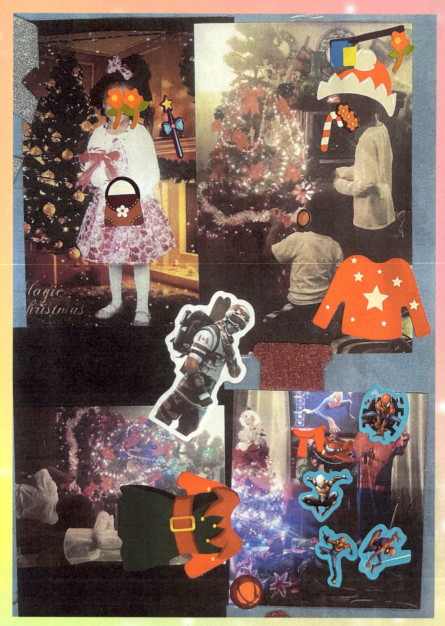

Christmas Time

Church

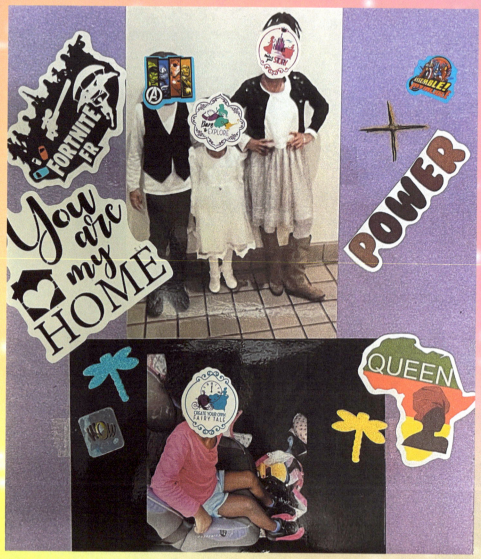

-A day of Blessing for Nia in church.
-Sisters day.

Do you have a sister or brother? Or do you have a cousin?

Cleaning

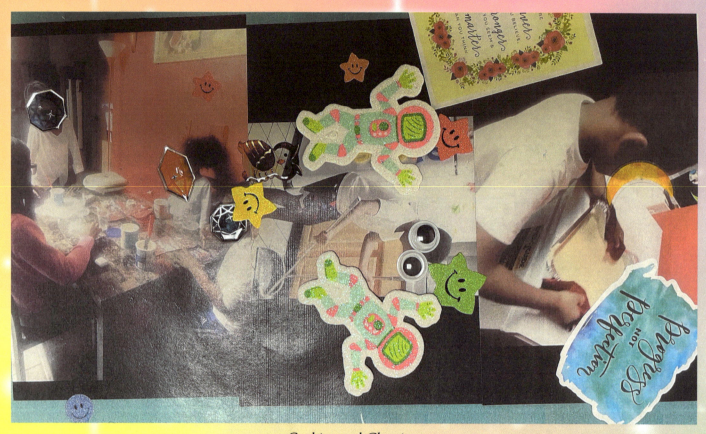

Cooking and Cleaning

We are making cupcakes

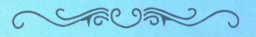

Dance

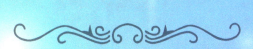

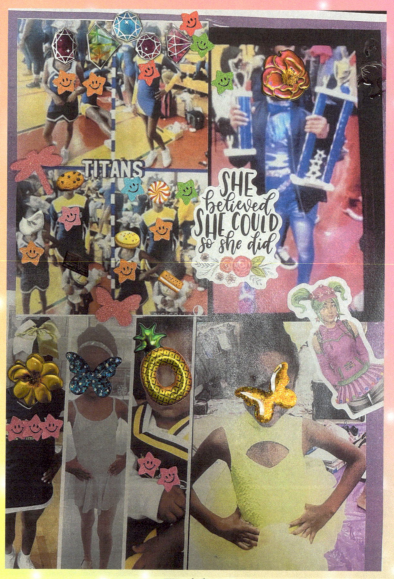

We did it!

Girls do you like doing this?

Family Time

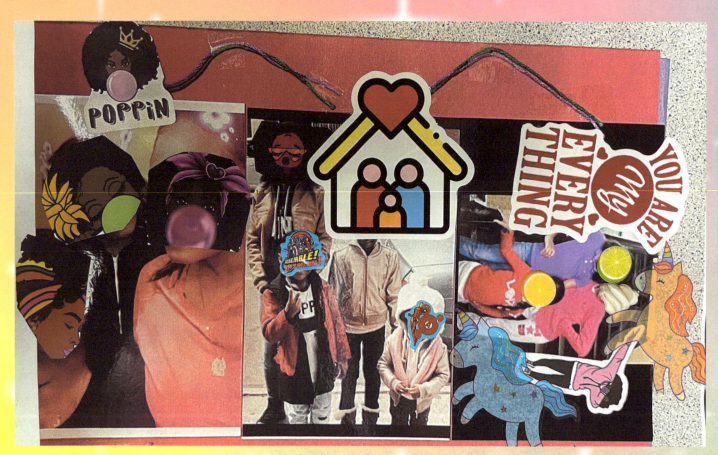

Just a day to take a picture.
Do you like taking pictures?

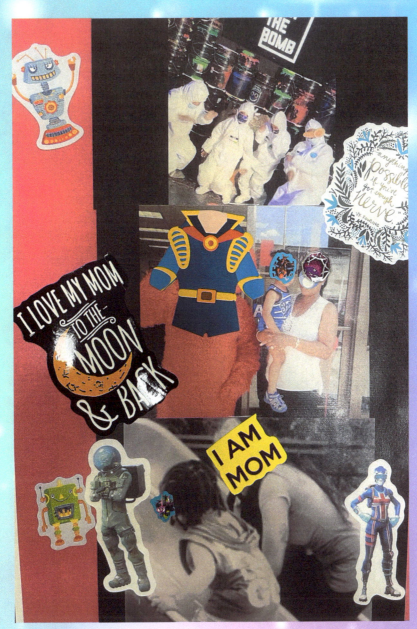

Do you like playing this?

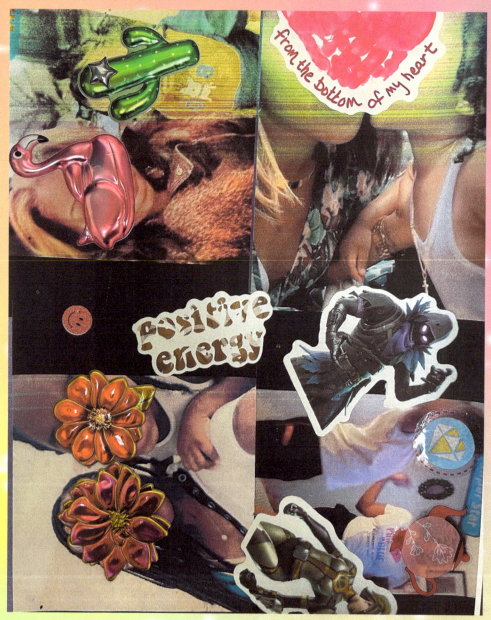

Mother and Son Day!

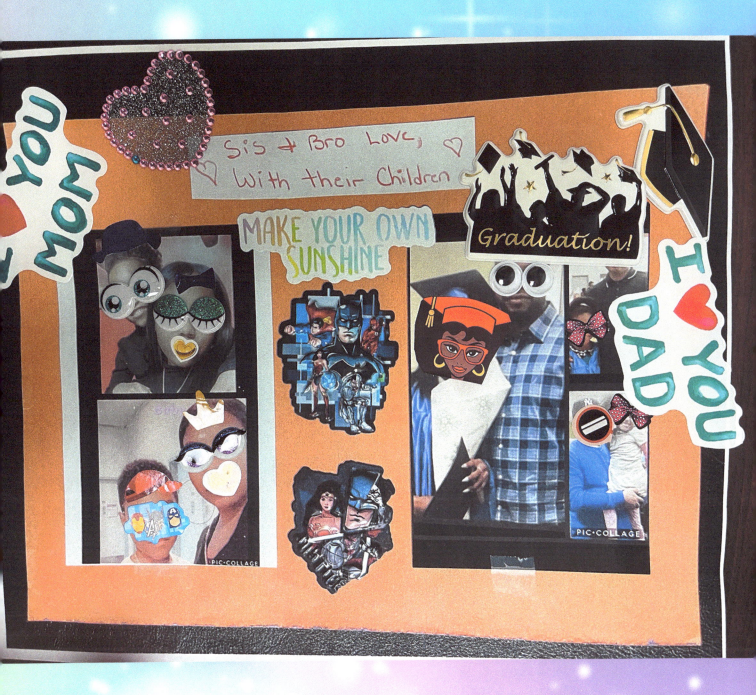

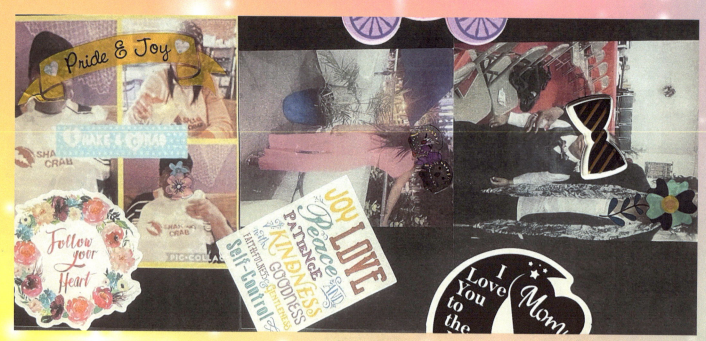

A great day with mom.
Do you like having mom time?

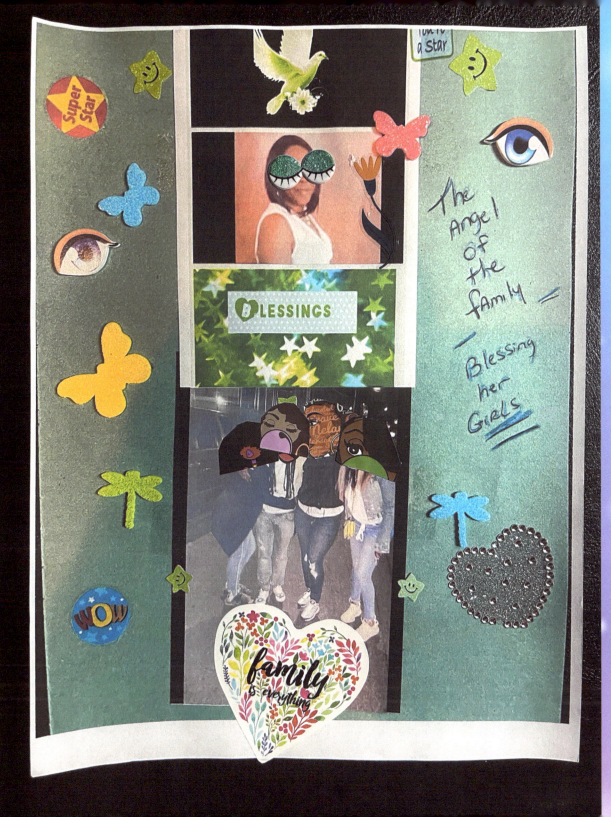

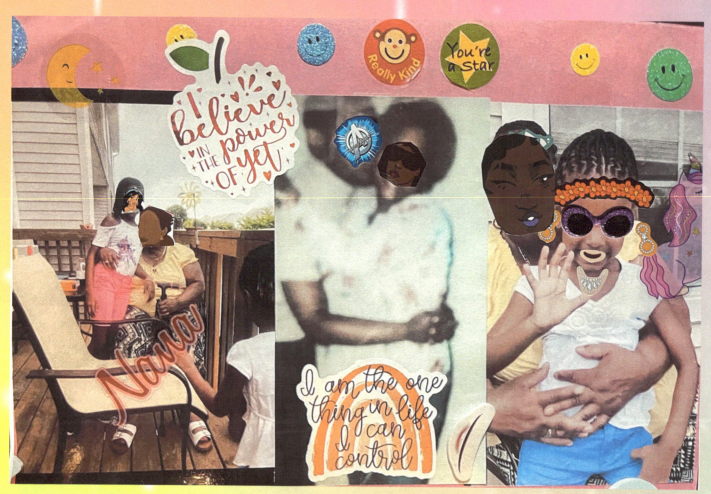

The joy with Nana and Son and Grands

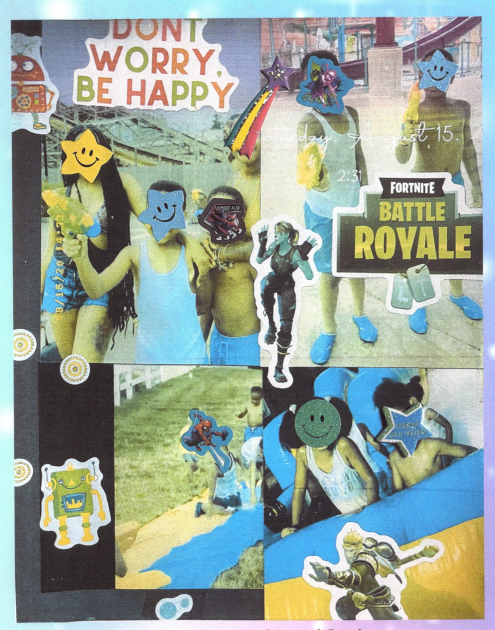

The joy with Nana and Son and Grands

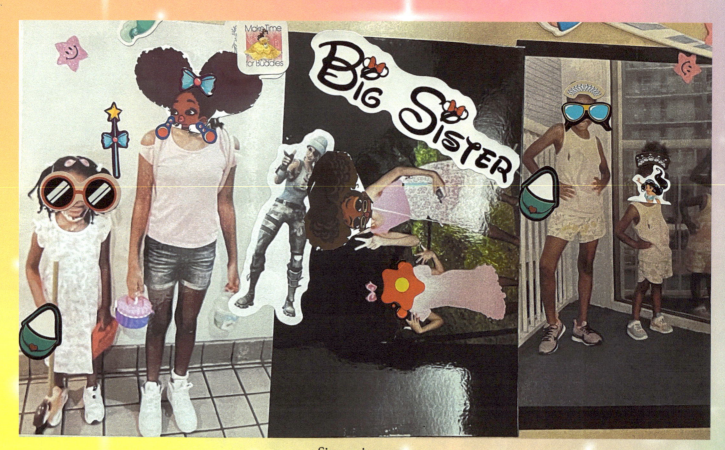

Sisters time out.
Do you have sisters or cousins?

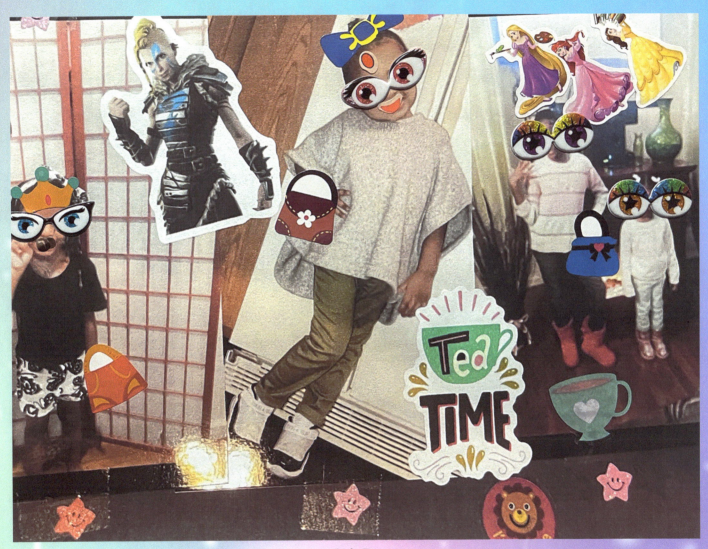
Girls Day

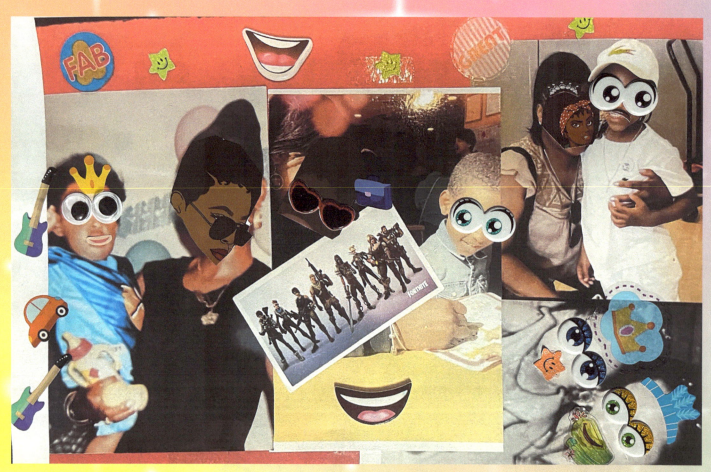

Ma & Auntie Time

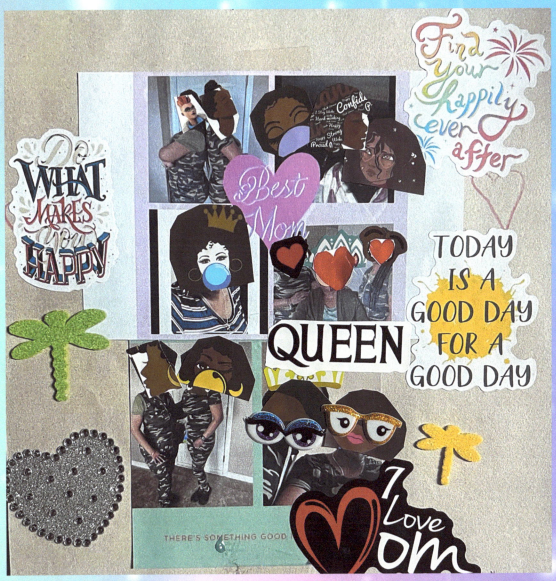

A great day with Mom!

Do you like having mom time?

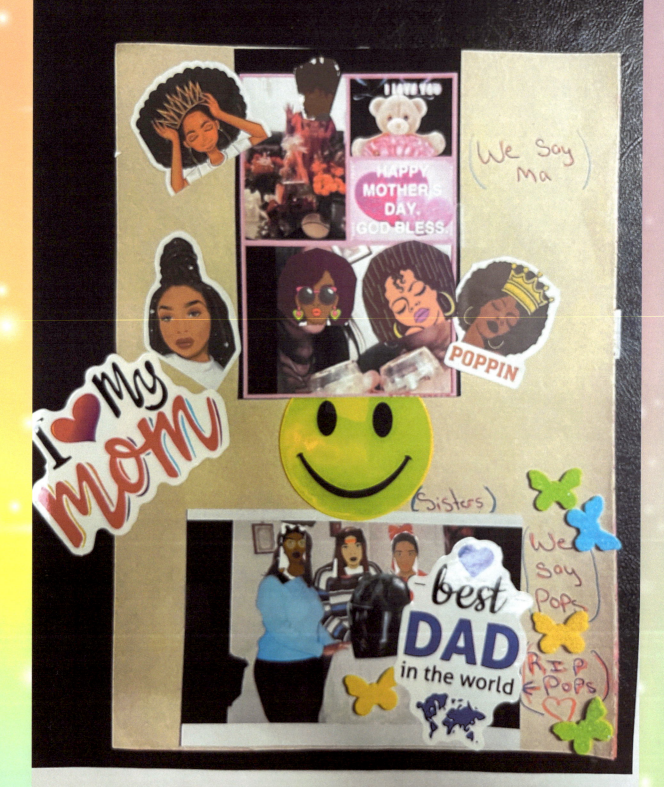

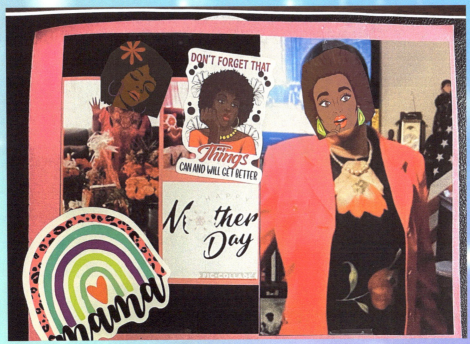

Ma and her girls.
We say Nana.

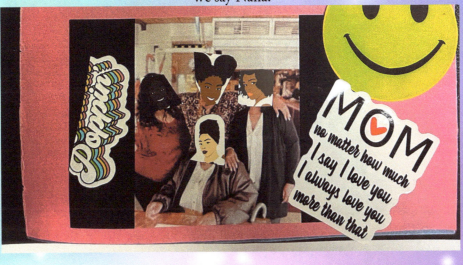

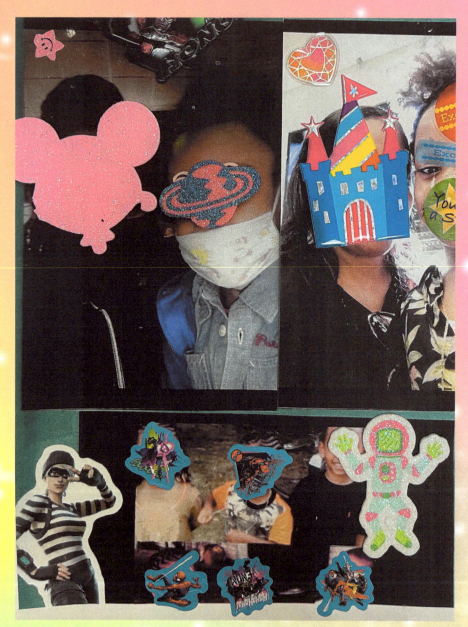

We love taking pictures with Grandma / Ma

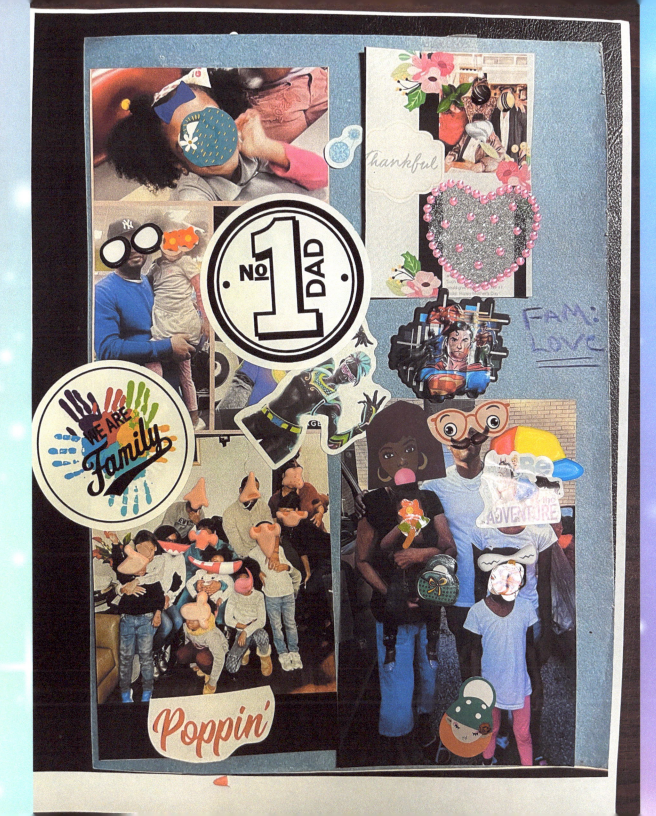

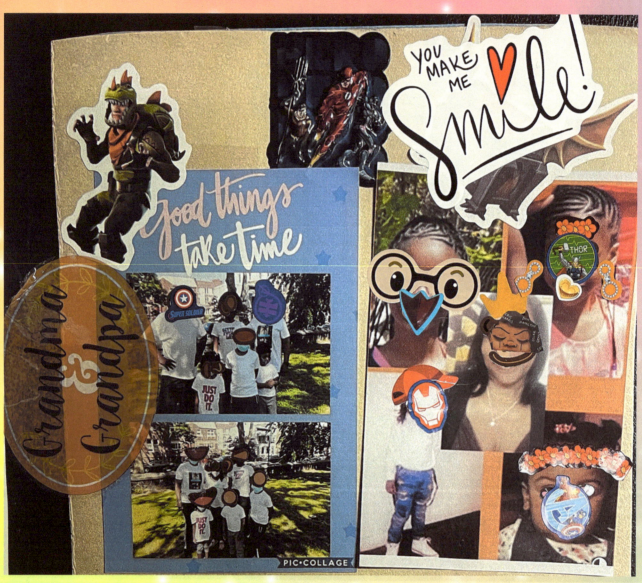

The Family Walk.

Grandma/Ma & Grands

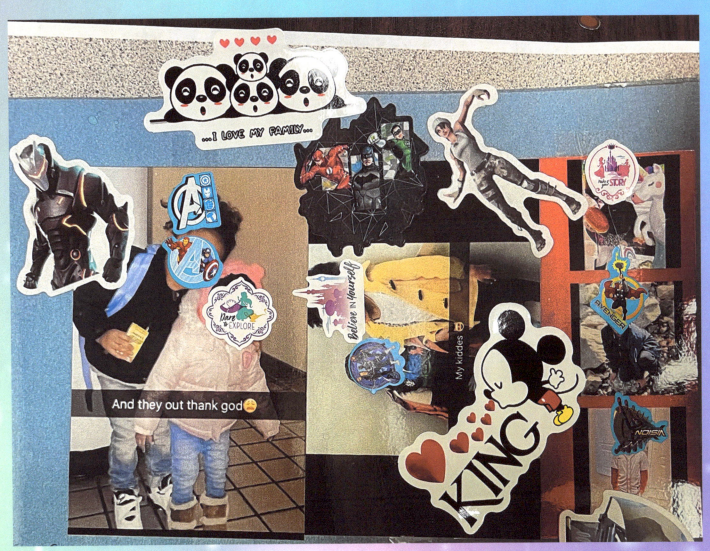

Cousin Time Makes our Day. Do you like cousin time?

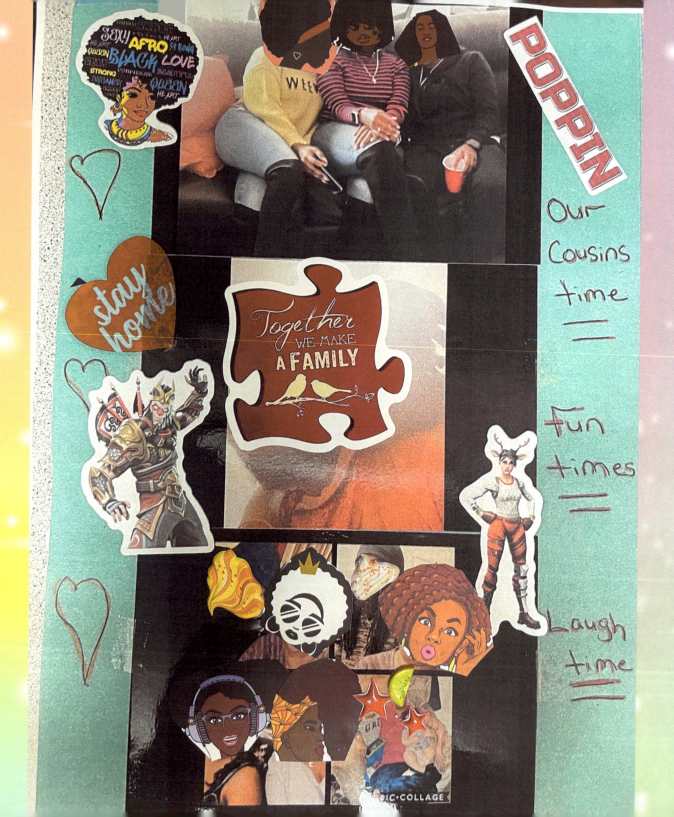

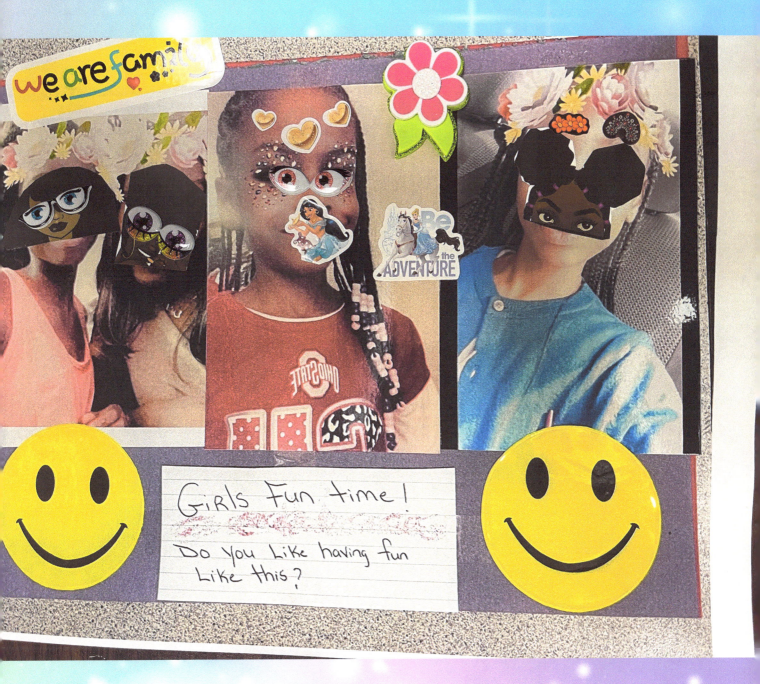

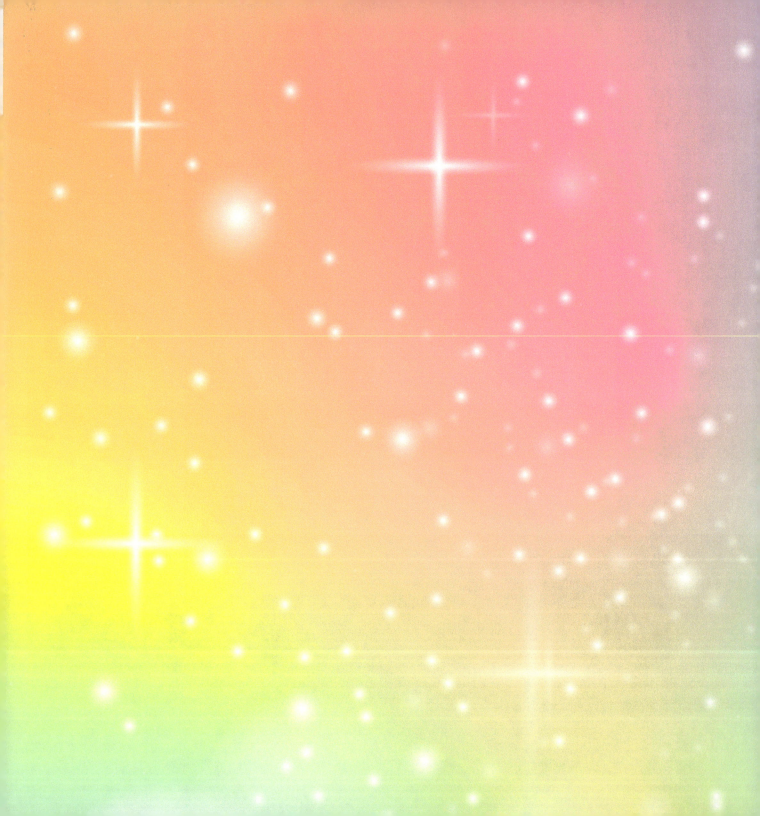

Playing

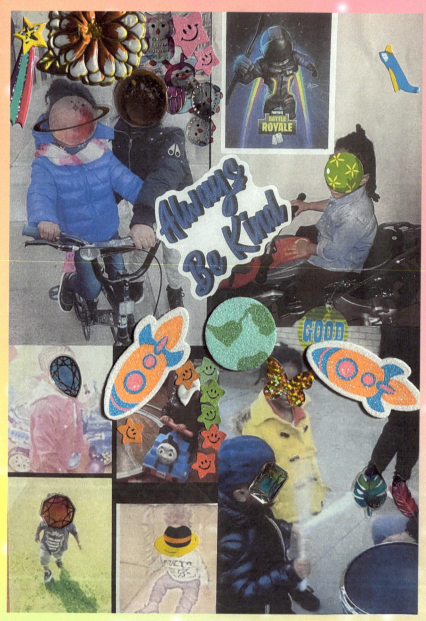

Outdoor and indoor fun!

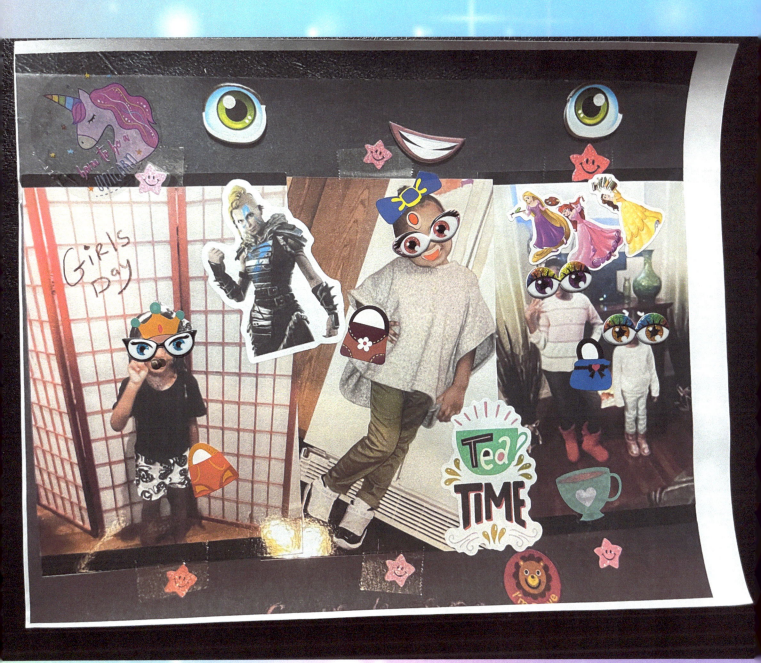

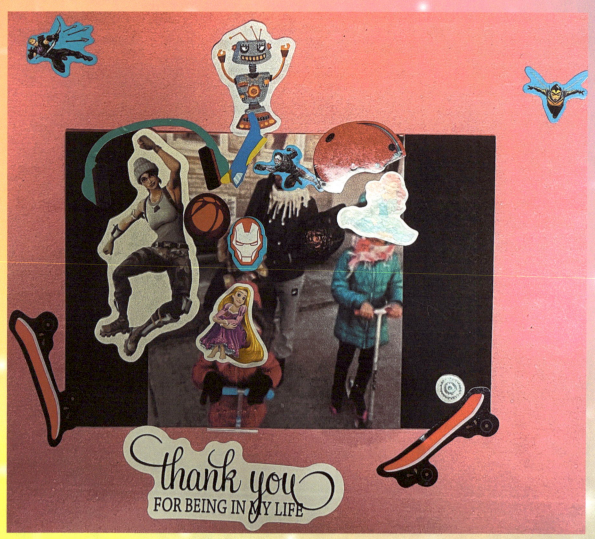

The entertainment with Children; indoor or outdoor.

Regardless of race, challenges or pandemic, make fun around the house with kids.

Also, the kids reflect on past experience of fun time to engage with peers.

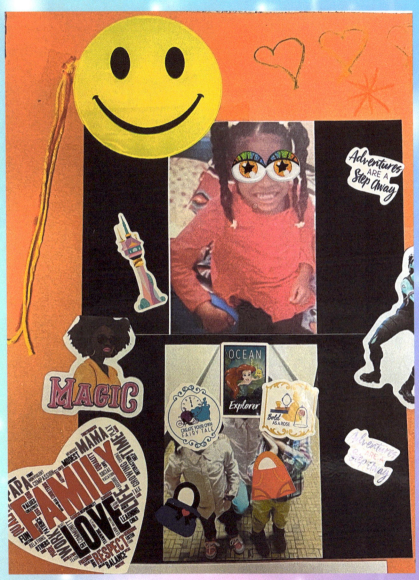

We love playing together (Sisters and cousins)

Do you like playing with your sisters or cousins?

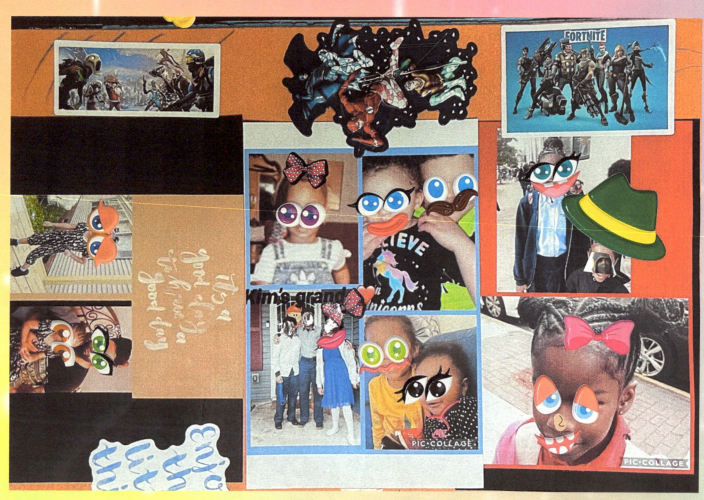

More cousin time

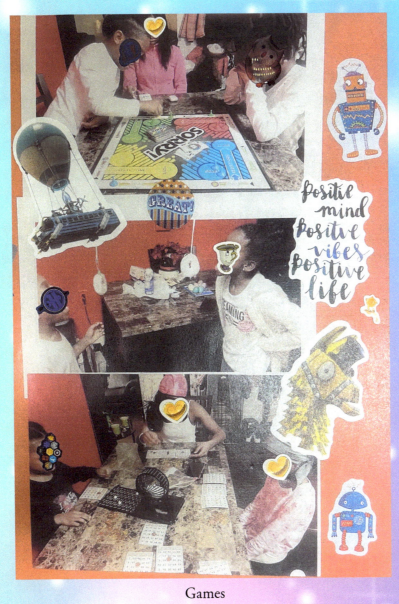

Games

Fun Time

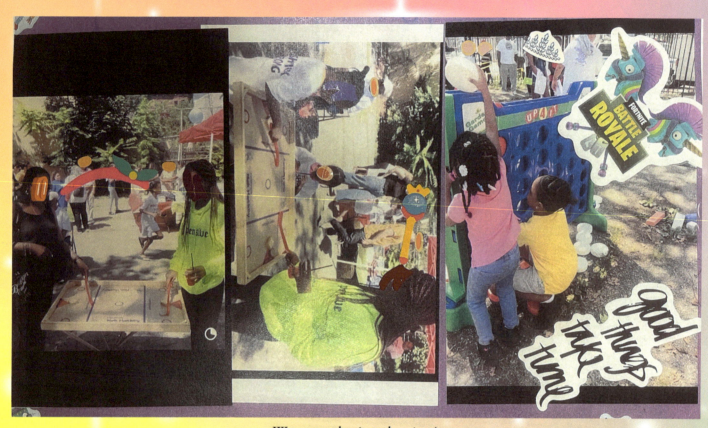

We are out having play time!

Do you like these games?

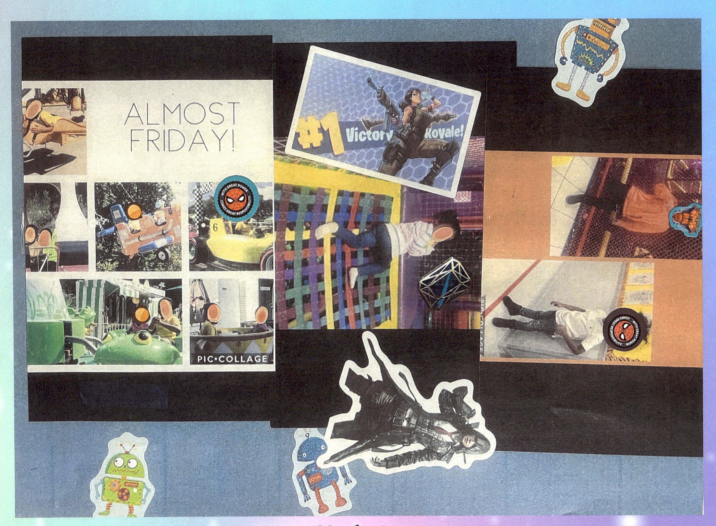
More fun time

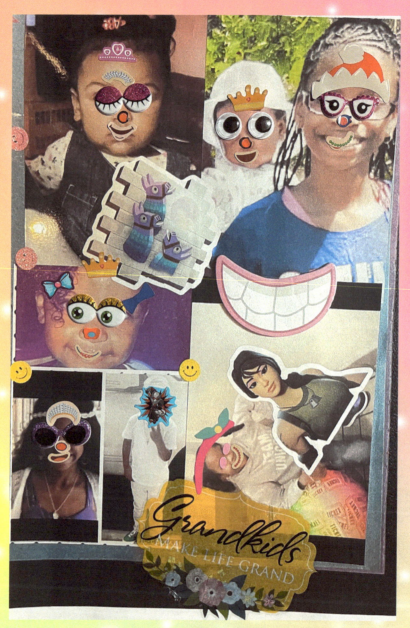

My grands smiling. Do you like to smile?

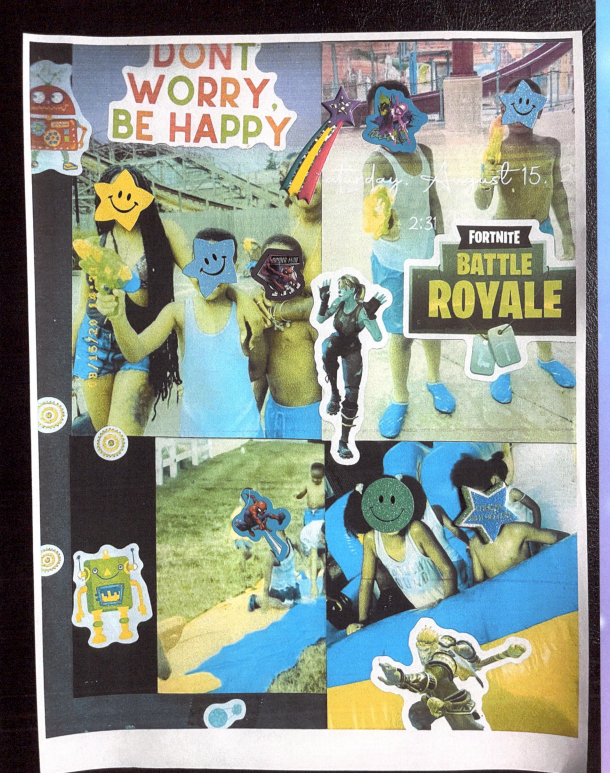

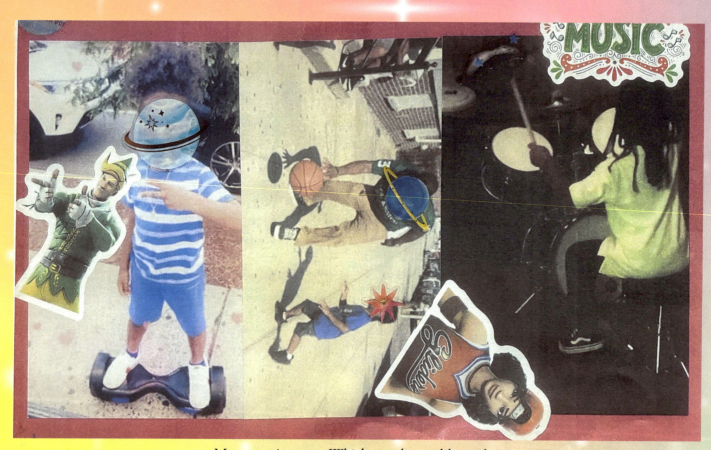

My entertainments. Which one do you like to do?

Going Out

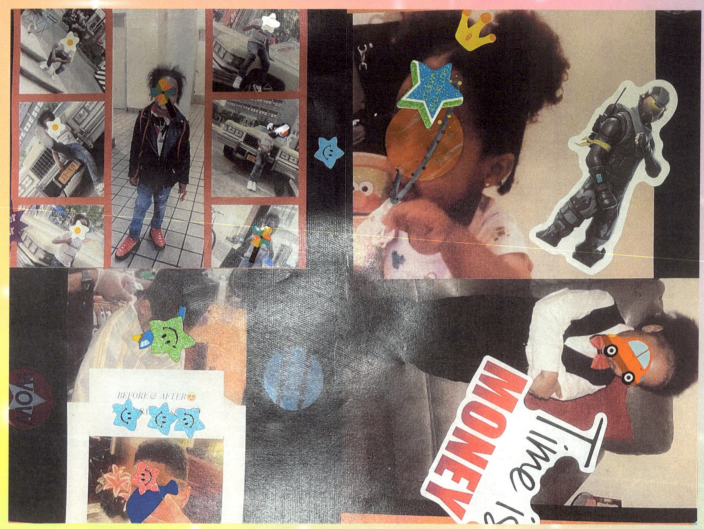

Before and After. Time for a haircut.

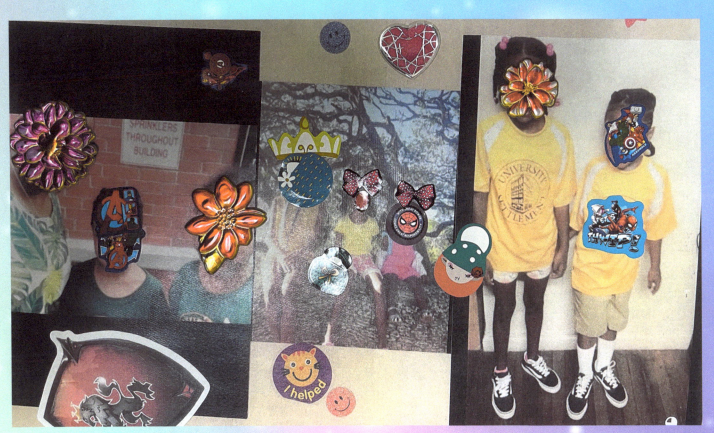

camp time/ summer time
Do you like the summer?

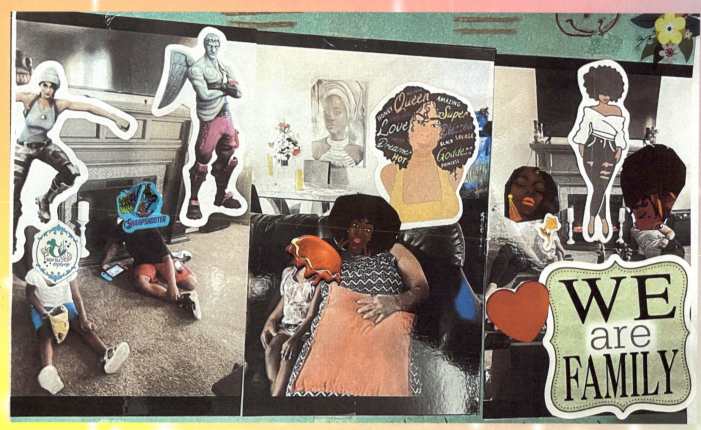

Fun around the house.

On vacation at my sister's/auntie's house.

Do you like going to your sister's house or friend's house?

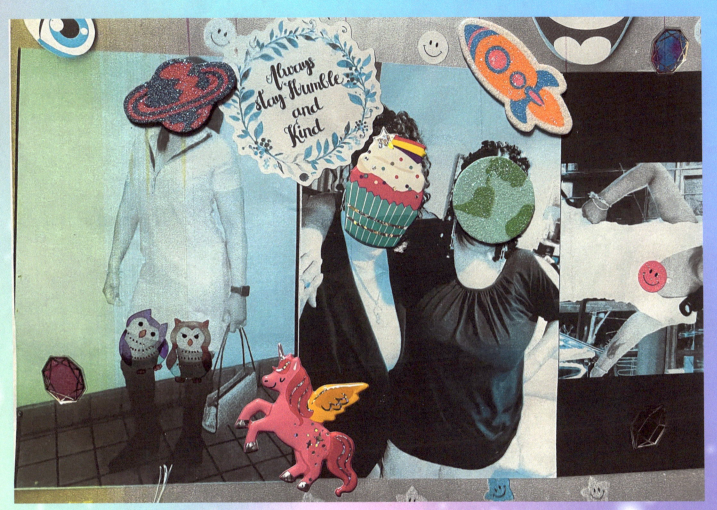

Sisters time out. Do you have sisters or cousins?

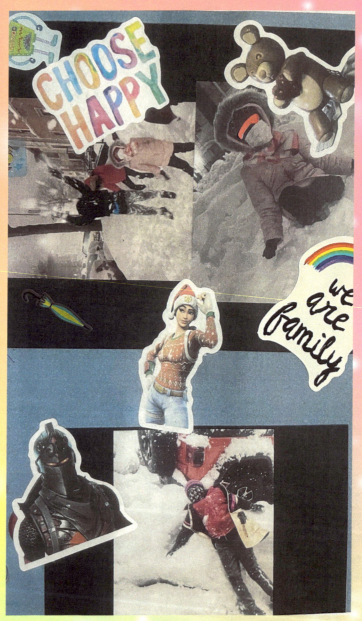

Our snow day. Do you like snow?

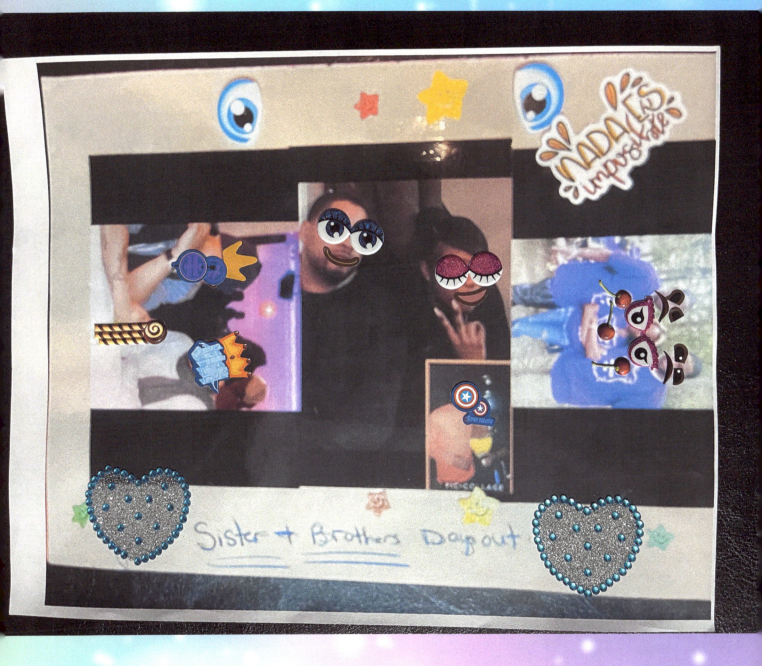

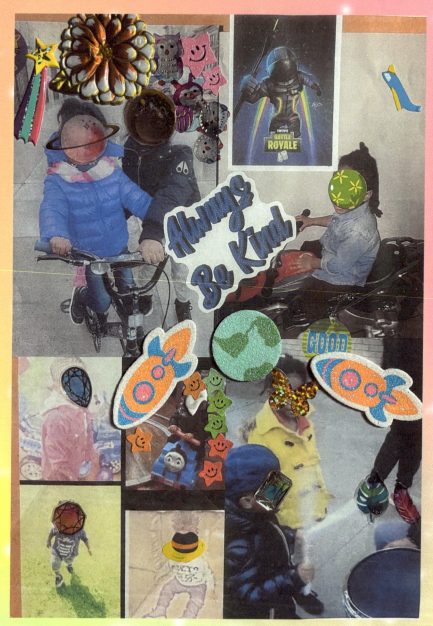

outdoor and indoor fun!

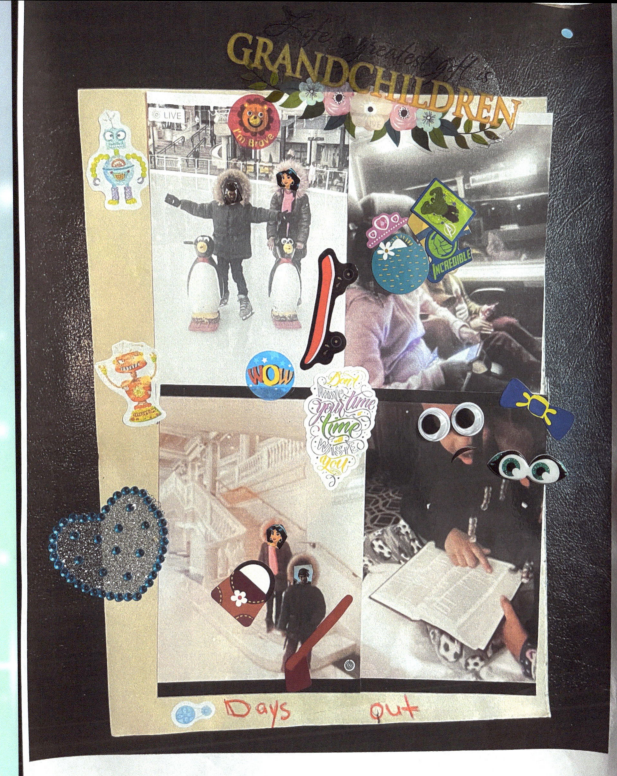

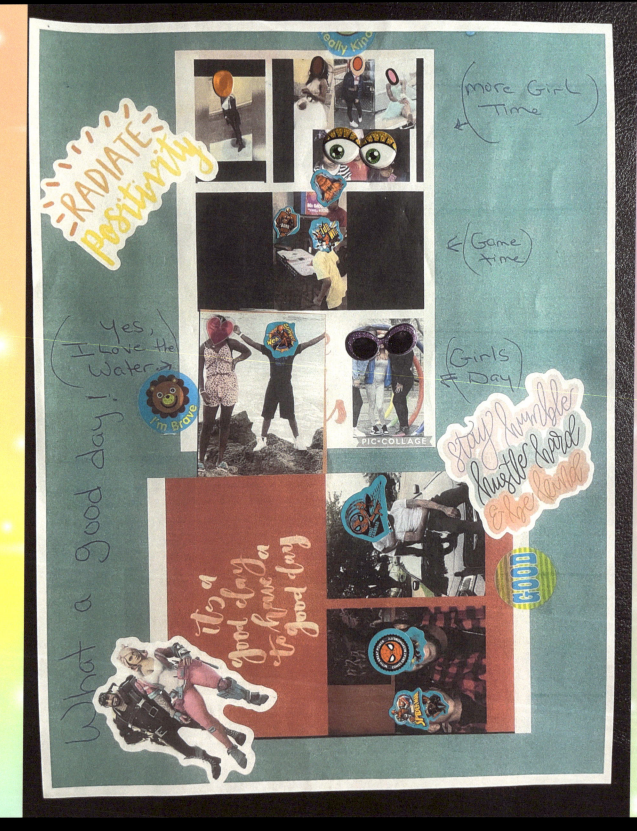

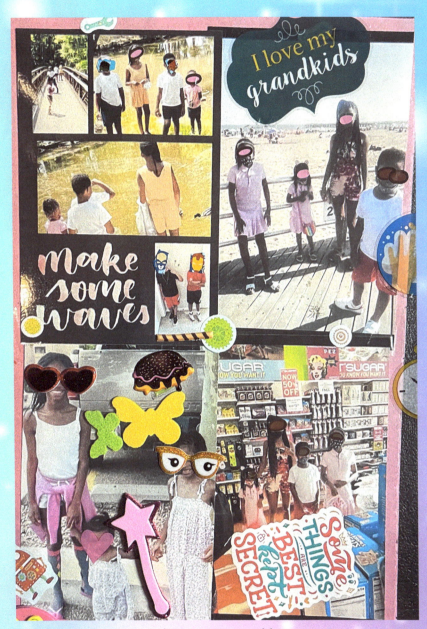

More great days out. Do you like going out?

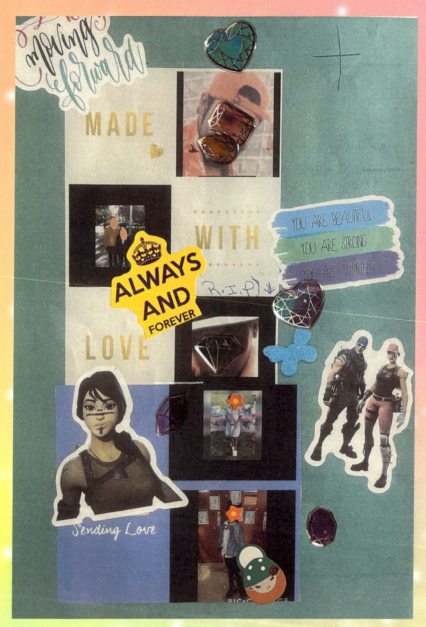

God children are a blessing.

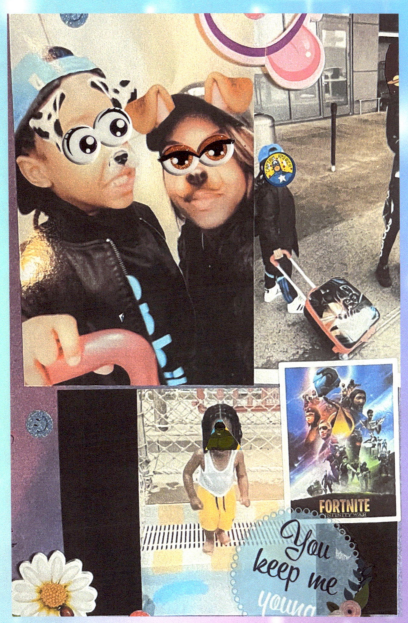

Traveling time for fun. Mom and Son. Do you like to travel?

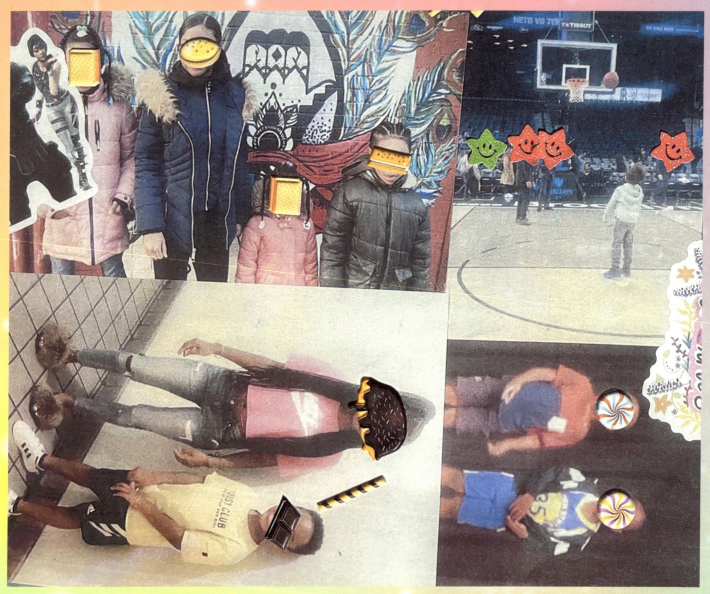

Can you guess what we are doing?

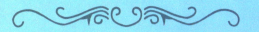

Graduation

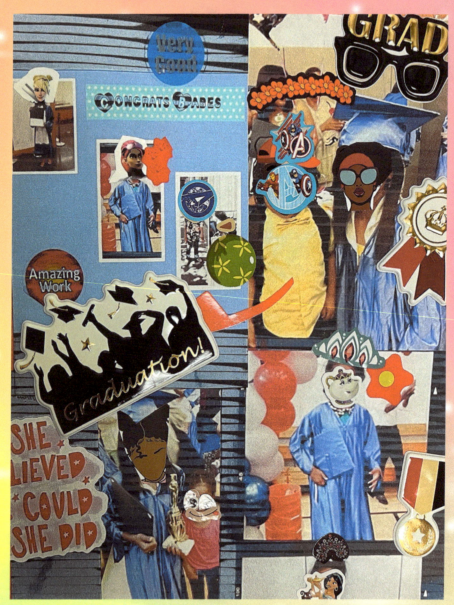

Graduation time for Grandson & Ma
Ya ya

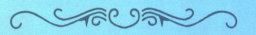

Halloween

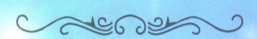

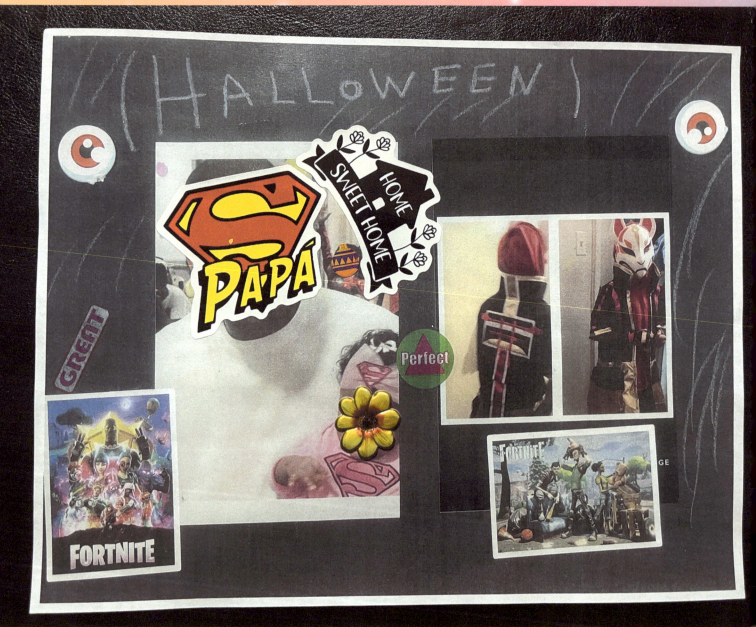

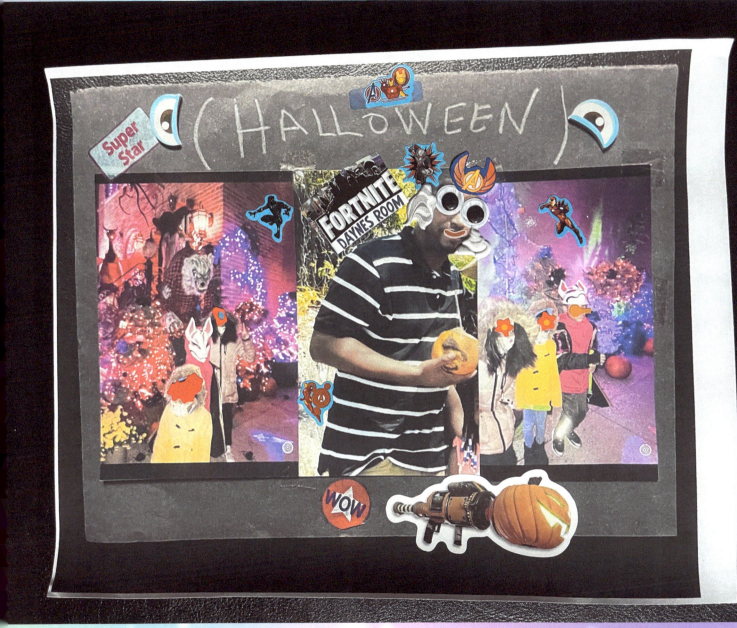

School

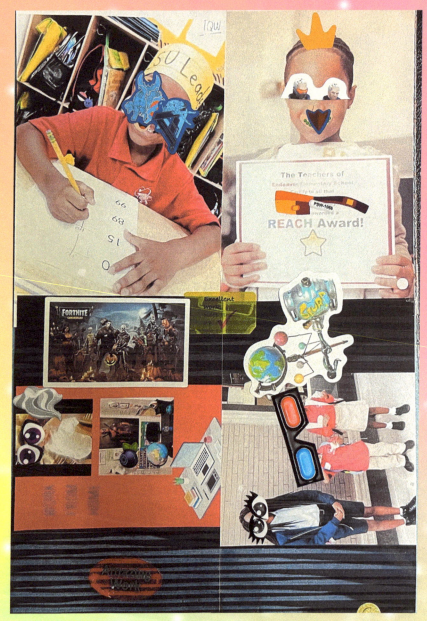

Working from home school and inside school.

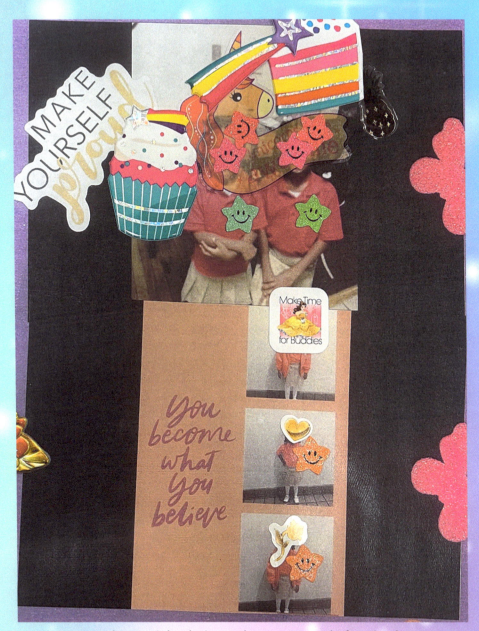

Heading to School. I'm ready. Are you ready for school?

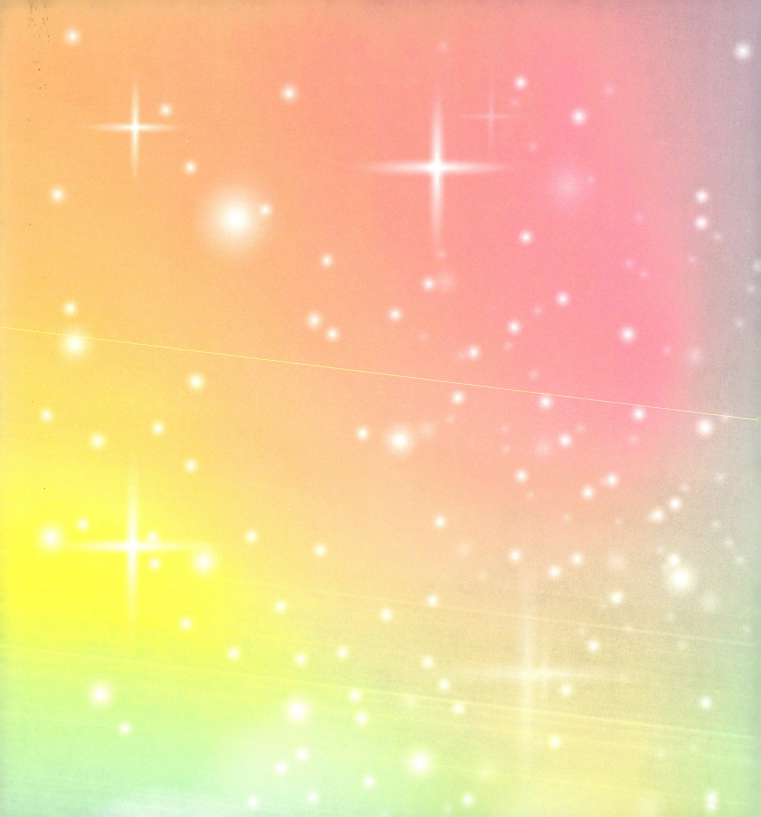

Our Beloved Family

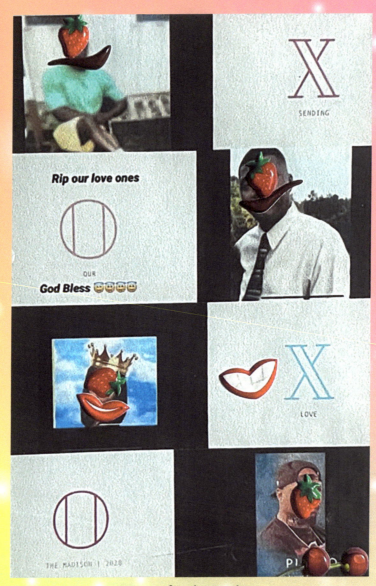

Rip our family members
We love y'all always.
Angels of the family.

The Moral to enjoyment is time

- Socialization skills

- Self reflection

- Self care

- Creativity Enhancement

- Emotional perspective

CPSIA information can be obtained
at www.ICGtesting.com
Printed in the USA
BVHW020346261021
619843BV00002B/11